THE ACTIVE SENIOR

A Guide to a Fit and Healthy Lifestyle

By

Dr Elizabeth M Harris

Copyright © by Dr. Elizabeth M Harris 2023.

TABLE OF CONTENT

INTRODUCTION

Exercise is essential for elderly persons (age 60+) seeing as physical fitness makes it easier to accomplish daily living functions (ADLs), including eating, taking a bath, toileting, dressing, getting into or out of a chair or a bed and moving around.

Exercise also increases muscular strength and bone density, which is particularly significant for women since they lose bone density quicker than males after menopause. Meanwhile, the heart and lung advantages of exercise assist enhance general health and counter some of the risks of chronic disease and illness.

Older individuals should exercise at least 2.5 to 5 hours of moderate-intensity aerobic activity per week, preferably spread over many days. Moderate-intensity aerobic exercises include brisk walking, cycling, swimming, dancing and nature hikes.

Walking: Walking is one of the finest forms of cardio for older folks and may be changed to fit the speed, distance or duration that works for the person. It takes strong balance but may be successful if one utilizes a cane or walker.

Cycling: Whether you ride an outdoor cycle or a stationary bike, cycling necessitates the activation of bigger muscles, especially the quadriceps and hamstrings, which results in higher blood flow and demands on the heart and lungs. As with other types of cardio, when this strain is repeated, the body adapts by improving its capacity to bear the extra load, thus the exercise helps the heart and lungs. Cycling is also a non-impact sport that may be good for anybody who wants to lessen ground reaction forces during exercise to aid with joint or muscle discomfort or dysfunction.

Dance: Whether you're performing Zumba, line dancing, or tango, moving your body (especially your hips) with non-stop dancing surely counts as cardio. Dancing not only boosts your heart rate, but also improves your balance, strengthens more significant muscle groups, and enhances your mood. Pair it with a partner or group for a social and physical exercise.

Nature Walks: Whether along a stream, beach, or mountain, nature walks may test your body's own proprioception or sense of self in space. Walking on various terrain helps increase strength, agility and balance for safer mobility overall. Spending time outside may also contribute to favorable psychological impacts, such as decreased anxiety and enhanced happiness.

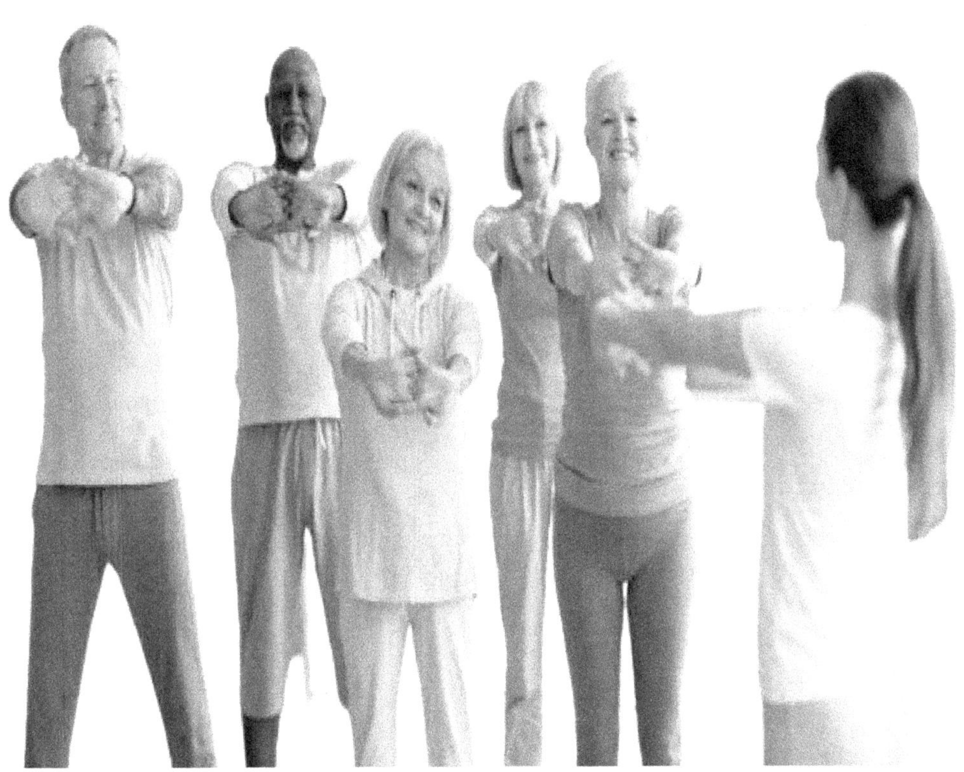

CHAPTER 1

Importance of Exercise for seniors

Exercise is crucial for seniors, as it plays a vital role in maintaining their physical, mental, and emotional health. The following are some of the reasons why exercise is essential for seniors:

1. **Improves Physical Health:** Regular exercise helps maintain flexibility, balance, strength, and mobility, all important factors for preventing falls and reducing the risk of injury.

2. **Boosts Mental Health:** Exercise has been shown to improve mood, reduce stress and anxiety, and boost self-esteem. This can lead to a better quality of life for seniors.

3. **Promotes Cognitive Function:** Exercise has been linked to a decrease in age-related cognitive decline and can improve memory and focus.

4. **Supports Independent Living:** Exercise can help seniors maintain their independence by maintaining their physical and mental function, allowing them to continue living without relying on others.

5. **Reduces Health Risks:** Exercise has been shown to reduce the risk of chronic conditions such as heart disease, stroke, diabetes, and certain types of cancer.

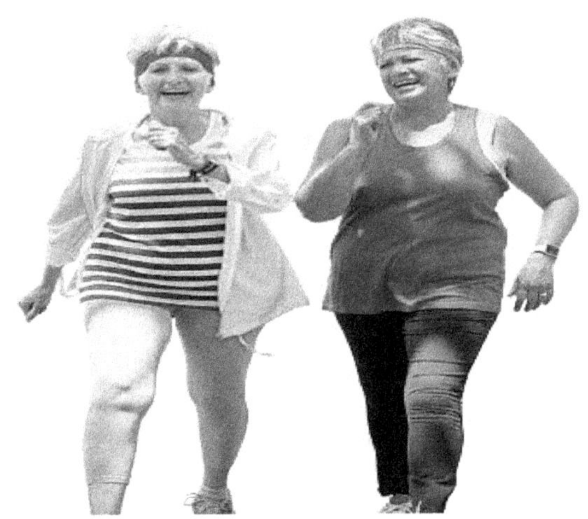

The benefits of exercise for seniors are numerous and can help improve their overall health and quality of life. Regular physical activity is essential for seniors to maintain their independence, improve physical and mental well-being, and reduce the risk of chronic health conditions.

The benefits of exercise for seniors are numerous and include the following:

1. **Improved Physical Health:** Regular exercise helps maintain flexibility, balance, strength, and mobility, all important factors for preventing falls and reducing the risk of injury. It can also help manage or improve arthritis, osteoporosis, and heart disease.

2. **Better Mental Health:** Exercise has been shown to improve mood, reduce stress and anxiety, and boost self-esteem. This can lead to a better quality of life for seniors.

3. **Increased Cognitive Function:** Exercise has been linked to a decrease in age-related cognitive decline and can improve memory and focus.

4. **Independent Living:** By maintaining physical and mental function, exercise can help seniors maintain their independence, allowing them to continue living without relying on others.

5. **Reduced Health Risks:** Exercise has been shown to reduce the risk of chronic conditions such as heart disease, stroke, diabetes, and certain types of cancer.

6. **Increased Energy and Endurance:** Regular exercise can improve cardiovascular health, increase energy levels, and reduce fatigue, making it easier for seniors to perform daily activities.

7. **Better Sleep:** Exercise has been linked to improved sleep patterns, helping seniors get a better night's rest.

8. **Improved Social Connection:** Exercise can allow seniors to connect with others and participate in social activities, helping to reduce feelings of isolation and loneliness.

Safety Considerations

When it comes to exercising, safety should always be a top priority, especially for seniors who may have physical limitations or chronic health conditions. The following are some safety considerations to keep in mind:

1. **Please consult with a healthcare provider:** Before starting any new exercise program, seniors should consult with their healthcare provider to ensure it is safe and appropriate for their health status.

2. **Start slow:** Seniors should start with low-impact exercises and gradually increase the intensity and duration of their workouts as they become fitter.

3. **Use proper form:** It is essential to use an appropriate format and technique when performing exercises to avoid injury and ensure that the activities are practical.

4. **Stay hydrated:** Exercise can cause dehydration, especially in warm weather, so it is essential to drink plenty of water before, during, and after exercise.

5. **Use proper equipment:** It is essential to use appropriate equipment, such as supportive footwear and joint braces, to reduce the risk of injury.

6. **Listen to your body:** Seniors should listen to their bodies and avoid overexerting themselves. If they experience any pain or discomfort, they should stop the exercise and seek medical attention if necessary.

7. **Warm-up and cool down:** It is essential to warm up before exercising to prepare the body for physical activity, and cool down after exercising, to help the body recover.

CHAPTER 2

Types of Workouts

Many different types of workouts can be suitable for seniors over 60. Some of the most common types include:

Aerobic Exercise

Aerobic exercise, also known as cardio exercise, is any physical activity that elevates the heart rate and improves the body's oxygen uptake. This exercise is essential for improving cardiovascular health, burning calories, and maintaining physical fitness. Aerobic exercise can be performed using various activities such as walking, running, cycling, swimming, and dancing.

During aerobic exercise, the body uses oxygen to produce energy, which can improve cardiovascular health by strengthening the heart and lungs. Additionally, regular aerobic exercise can help control weight, reduce the risk of chronic health conditions such as heart disease, stroke, and type 2 diabetes, and improve mental health by reducing stress and anxiety.

To achieve the health benefits of aerobic exercise, it is recommended that seniors engage in at least 150 minutes of moderate-intensity aerobic activity per week, or 30 minutes per day for at least five days per week. It is essential to start slowly and gradually increase the intensity and duration of aerobic exercise to avoid overexertion and injury.

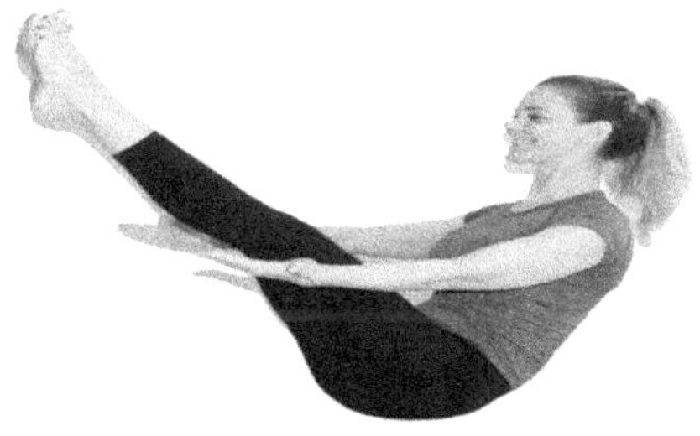

Strength Training

Strength training, also known as resistance training, involves the use of weights or resistance bands to build muscle and increase strength. This exercise is essential for seniors as it can help maintain and improve muscle mass, which can decline with age.

Strength training exercises typically involve lifting weights or performing resistance exercises against resistance, such as push-ups, squats, and bicep curls. This type of exercise can help build muscle and increase strength, improving physical function, reducing the risk of falls, and improving overall physical and mental health.

Strength training should be performed twice weekly, with one to two sets of 8–12 repetitions for each exercise. To avoid injury and overexertion, it is essential to start with lighter weights and gradually increase the weight as strength improves.

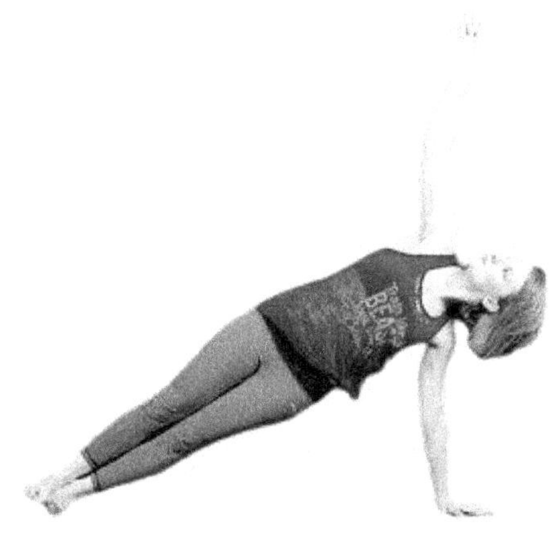

Balance and Flexibility

Balance and flexibility are essential components of physical fitness that are crucial for overall health and wellness, especially for seniors over 60. These components can decline with age, increasing the risk of falls and injury.

Balance exercises are designed to improve stability and reduce the risk of falls. Examples of balance exercises include standing on one foot, walking heel to toe, and using a balance board. Regular balance training can help improve stability, reduce the risk of falls, and maintain independence and quality of life.

Flexibility exercises are designed to improve the range of motion and reduce muscle stiffness. Examples of flexibility exercises include stretching, yoga, and tai chi. Regular flexibility training can improve the content of the action, decrease muscle stiffness, and enhance physical and mental well-being.

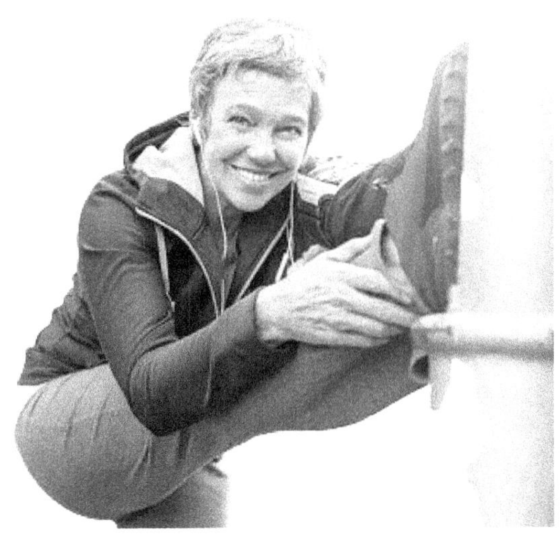

Seniors need to consult a doctor or physical therapist before starting a new exercise program to determine what exercises are appropriate for their needs and fitness level. It is also essential to start slow and gradually increase the intensity and duration of exercises to avoid overexertion and injury.

Low-Impact Workouts

Low-impact workouts are gentler physical activities on the joints and bones, making them an excellent option for seniors and people with joint pain or injury. These workouts can provide many of the same health benefits as high-impact workouts but with less risk of injury or strain on the joints.

Examples of low-impact workouts include walking, swimming, cycling, yoga, tai chi, and water aerobics. These exercises are low-impact because they place less stress on the joints and bones, reducing the risk of injury and making them ideal for seniors and people with joint pain or injury.

Low-impact workouts can provide many of the same health benefits as high-impact workouts, such as improving cardiovascular health, burning calories, and reducing the risk of chronic health conditions such as heart disease, stroke, and type 2 diabetes. Low-impact workouts can also improve mental health by reducing stress and anxiety.

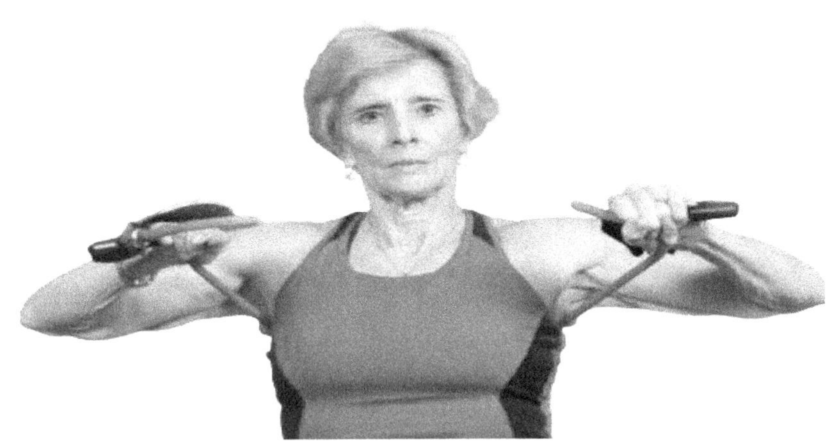

Water Exercise

Water exercise, also known as aquatic exercise, is a type of physical activity performed in water. This exercise is ideal for seniors as it provides a gentle, low-impact workout on the joints yet provides many of the same health benefits as high-impact workouts.

Water exercise can include swimming, aerobics, water walking, and water resistance training. The water's resistance helps improve cardiovascular health, build strength, and increase flexibility. The water's buoyancy also helps reduce stress on the joints, making it an ideal option for seniors and people with joint pain or injuries.

Water exercise is often performed in a pool or other aquatic setting and can be adapted to suit a wide range of fitness levels and abilities. It is essential to consult with a doctor or physical therapist before starting a new exercise program to determine what exercises are appropriate for your individual needs and fitness level.

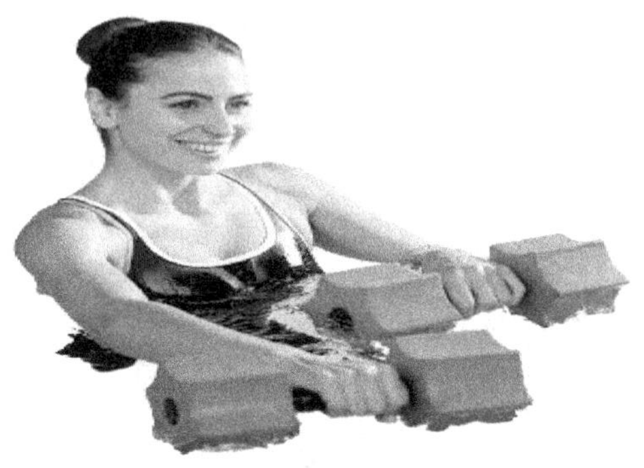

Water Exercise

Yoga and Pilates

Yoga and Pilates are two types of physical activity that have become increasingly popular among seniors in recent years. Both practices focus on body control, flexibility, and strength, making them ideal for seniors looking to improve their overall physical health and well-being.

Yoga is a practice that has been used for thousands of years to promote physical, mental, and emotional well-being. It involves a series of poses and movements designed to improve flexibility, build strength, and reduce stress. Yoga is low-impact, making it an ideal option for seniors and people with joint pain or injuries.

Pilates is a type of exercise focusing on building core strength, improving posture, and increasing flexibility. It involves a series of controlled movements designed to challenge the body and improve overall physical health. Pilates is also low-impact, making it an ideal option for seniors and people with joint pain or injury.

Yoga and Pilates can be performed in class or at home using instructional videos or books. It is essential to consult with a doctor or physical therapist before starting a new exercise program to determine what exercises are appropriate for your individual needs and fitness level.

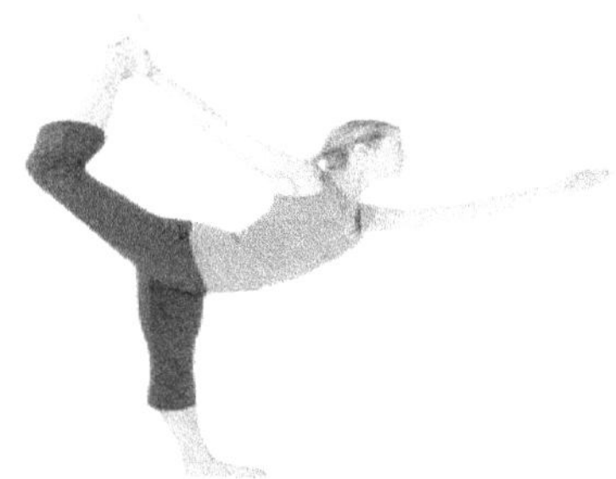

Many different types of workouts are suitable for seniors over 60. Choosing an exercise program appropriate for the individual's physical abilities, interests, and health status are essential. Regular exercise is necessary to maintain physical, mental, and emotional health and improve the overall quality of life.

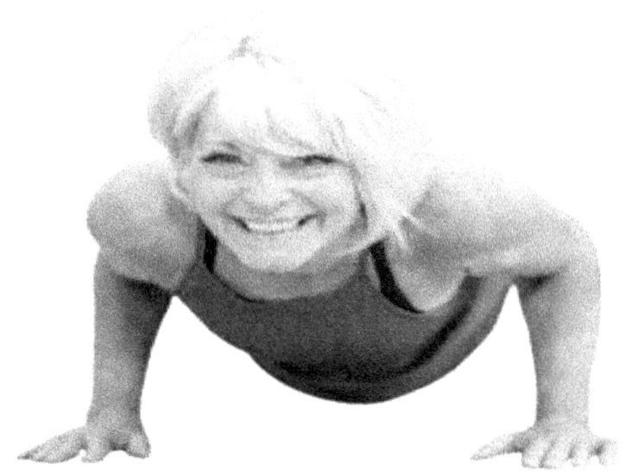

CHAPTER 3

Workout Routines

Beginner Workouts

Beginner workouts are a set of exercises designed specifically for people who are new to physical activity or who have not exercised regularly in some time. They are a great way for seniors to start incorporating physical activity into their daily routine and improve their physical health and well-being. A typical beginner workout for seniors may include:

1. **Gentle aerobic exercise:** Gentle aerobic exercise, such as walking or swimming, is a great way for seniors to get their heart rate up and improve their cardiovascular health.

2. **Gentle strength training:** Gentle strength training exercises, such as resistance band exercises or light weightlifting, can help seniors build and maintain muscle mass.

3. **Gentle balance and flexibility exercises:** Gentle balance and flexibility exercises, such as yoga or tai chi, can help seniors improve their balance and flexibility, reducing the risk of falls and injury.

4. **Low-impact workouts:** Low-impact workouts, such as water aerobics or water walking, are gentler on the joints and bones, making them a great option for seniors and people with joint pain or injury.

It is important to start slowly and gradually increase the intensity and duration of your workouts over time. It is also important to consult with a doctor or physical therapist before starting a new workout routine to determine what exercises are appropriate for your individual needs and fitness level.

Intermediate workouts are a set of exercises designed for individuals who have a moderate level of fitness and have been regularly participating in physical activity for some time. They are designed to challenge individuals and help them improve their physical health and well-being.

A typical intermediate workout for seniors may include:

1. **Moderate-intensity aerobic exercise:** Moderate-intensity aerobic exercise, such as brisk walking, jogging, cycling, or swimming, is a great way to challenge individuals and improve cardiovascular health.
2. **Strength training:** Strength training exercises, such as weightlifting, resistance band exercises, or bodyweight exercises, can help individuals build and maintain muscle mass.
3. **Balance and flexibility exercises:** Balance and flexibility exercises, such as yoga or tai chi, can help improve balance and flexibility, reducing the risk of falls and injury.
4. **Low-impact workouts:** Low-impact workouts, such as water aerobics or water walking, can help individuals maintain their physical health and well-being without putting too much stress on their joints and bones.

It is important to listen to your body and gradually increase the intensity and duration of your workouts over time. It is also important to consult with a doctor or physical therapist before starting a new workout routine to determine what exercises are appropriate for your individual needs and fitness level.

Advanced Workouts

Advanced workouts are a set of exercises designed for individuals who have a high level of fitness and have been regularly participating in physical activity for a long time. They are designed to push individuals to their limits and help them achieve their fitness goals.

A typical advanced workout for seniors may include:

1. **High-intensity aerobic exercise:** High-intensity aerobic exercise, such as running, cycling, or swimming, can help individuals challenge themselves and improve their cardiovascular health.

2. **Intense strength training:** Intense strength training exercises, such as heavy weightlifting or resistance band exercises, can help individuals build and maintain muscle mass and strength.

3. **Balance and flexibility exercises:** Balance and flexibility exercises, such as yoga or tai chi, can help improve balance and flexibility, reducing the risk of falls and injury.

4. **High-impact workouts:** High-impact workouts, such as jumping jacks or jumping rope, can help individuals challenge themselves and improve their overall physical health and well-being.

Customized workouts are exercise routines that are tailored to meet the specific needs, goals, and abilities of individuals. They take into account an individual's current fitness level, health status, and personal goals to create a workout routine that is safe, effective, and achievable.

Customized workouts for seniors may include a combination of aerobic exercise, strength training, balance and flexibility exercises, low-impact workouts, and water exercise, among others. The exercises included in a customized workout routine may also be adjusted based on the individual's level of experience, physical ability, and any medical conditions they may have.

For seniors, customized workouts can help improve their overall physical health and well-being and reduce the risk of falls and injury. They can also help individuals achieve their fitness goals and improve their quality of life.

It is important to work with a qualified personal trainer or physical therapist to create a customized workout routine that meets your individual needs and goals. A professional can help you determine what exercises are appropriate for your fitness level, provide proper form and technique instruction, and help you stay safe and injury-free while working out.

CHAPTER 4

Equipment and Gear

Equipment and gear are essential for safe and effective workouts. For seniors, the right equipment and gear can help reduce the risk of injury, improve workout performance, and enhance overall physical health and well-being. Some common types of equipment and gear for seniors include:

Essential Equipment

Essential equipment is a type of gear that is required to perform a workout safely and effectively. For seniors, essential equipment can help reduce the risk of injury, improve workout performance, and enhance overall physical health and well-being. Some essential equipment for seniors include:

1. **Exercise mats:** Exercise mats provide a cushioned surface for exercises, such as yoga or Pilates. They can help reduce the risk of injury and provide comfort during workouts.

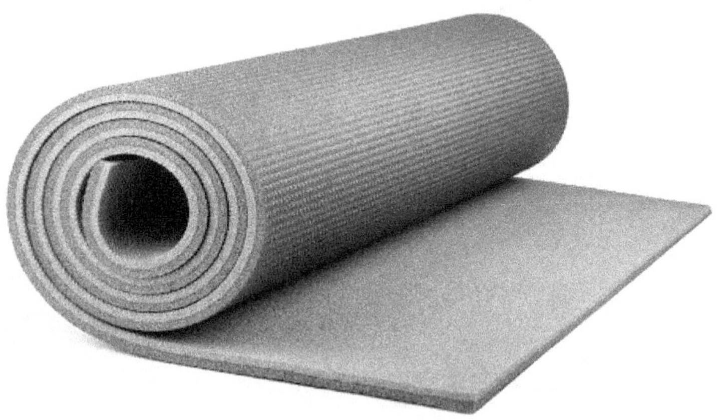

2. **Resistance bands:** Resistance bands are used for strength training exercises, such as arm and leg extensions. They can help improve muscle tone and strength without the need for heavy weights.

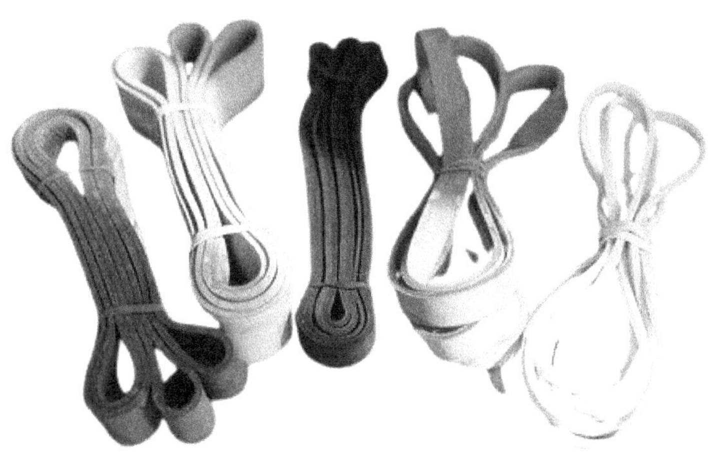

3. **Hand weights:** Hand weights, such as dumbbells, are used for strength training exercises, such as bicep curls or shoulder presses. They come in a variety of weights and can be adjusted based on an individual's fitness level.

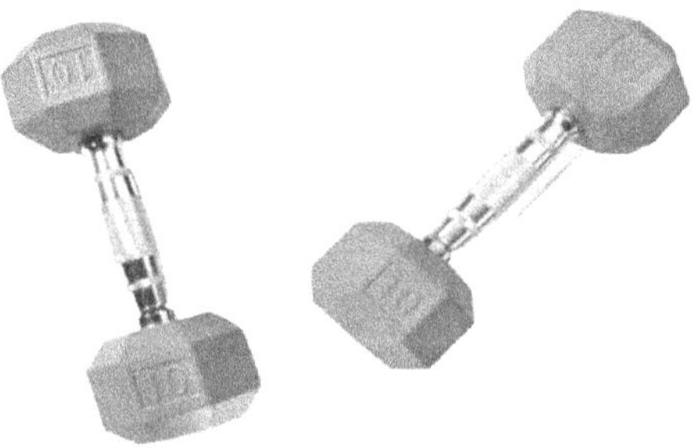

4. **Stability balls:** stability balls are used for balance and core stability exercises. They can help improve balance, stability, and coordination.

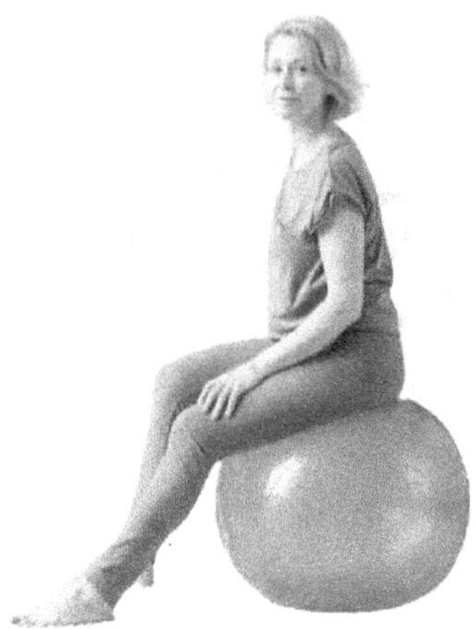

5. **Comfortable clothing:** Comfortable clothing, such as sweat-wicking fabric, is important for keeping seniors comfortable and dry during workouts.

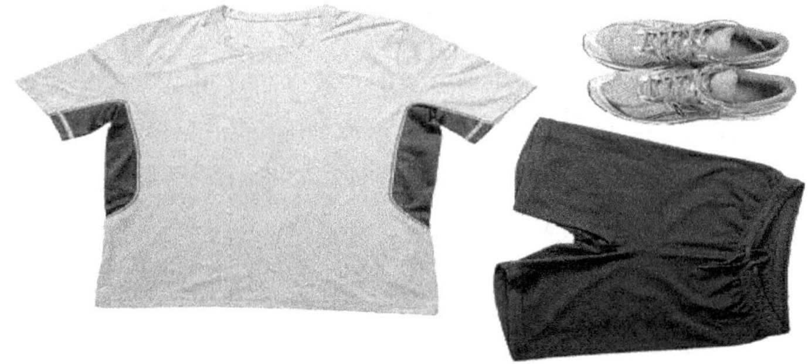

It is important to choose essential equipment that is appropriate for your fitness level, health status, and personal goals. It is also important to consult with a doctor or physical therapist before starting a new workout routine to determine what essential equipment is appropriate for your individual needs.

Recommended Gear

Recommended gear is equipment that is not essential, but is recommended for optimal performance and comfort during workouts. For seniors, recommended gear can enhance overall workout experience, provide additional support and comfort, and reduce the risk of injury. Some recommended gear for seniors include:

1. **Exercise gloves:** Exercise gloves can help protect seniors' hands from blisters and calluses, and provide a comfortable grip during strength training exercises.

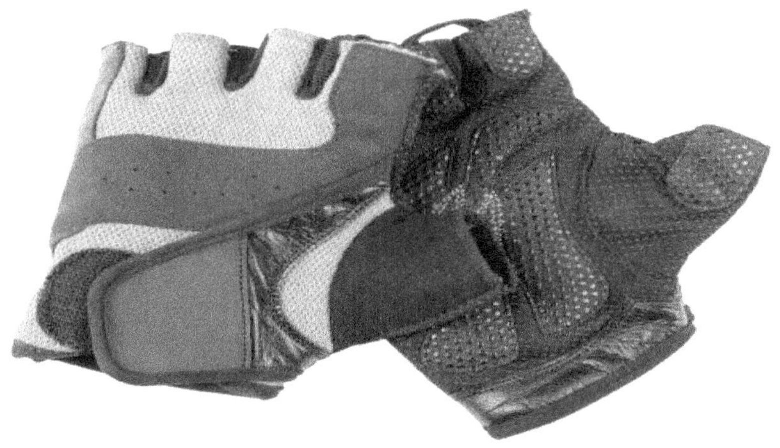

2. **Exercise shoes:** Exercise shoes provide support, stability, and cushioning for seniors during workouts. They can help prevent injuries and improve overall workout performance.

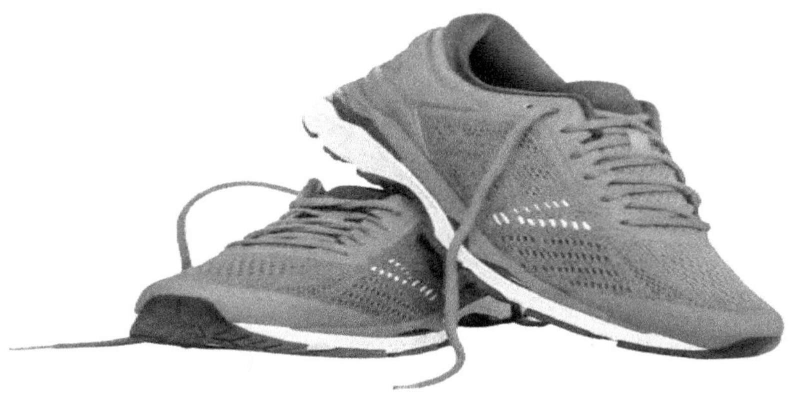

3. **Heart rate monitor:** A heart rate monitor is a device that measures the heart rate during physical activity. This can help seniors monitor their intensity levels and ensure that they are working within their target heart rate zone.

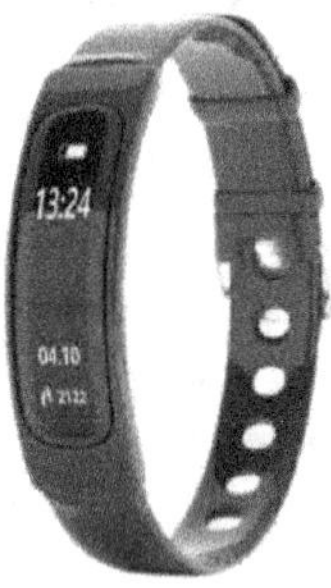

4. **Foam rollers:** Foam rollers are used for foam rolling, a type of self-massage that can help improve muscle recovery, flexibility, and reduce muscle soreness.

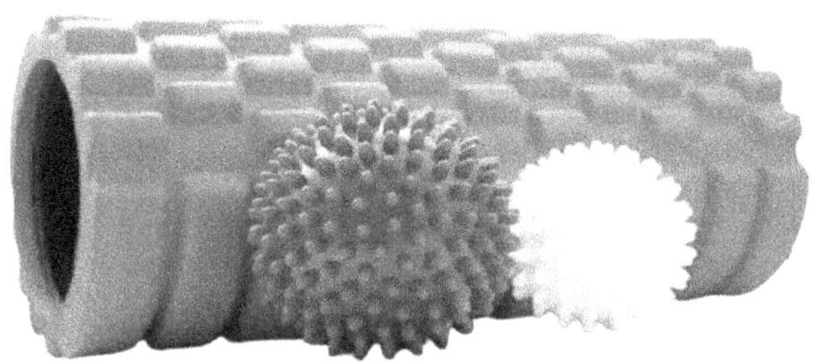

5. **Athletic tape:** Athletic tape can be used to provide support and stability for joints during physical activity.

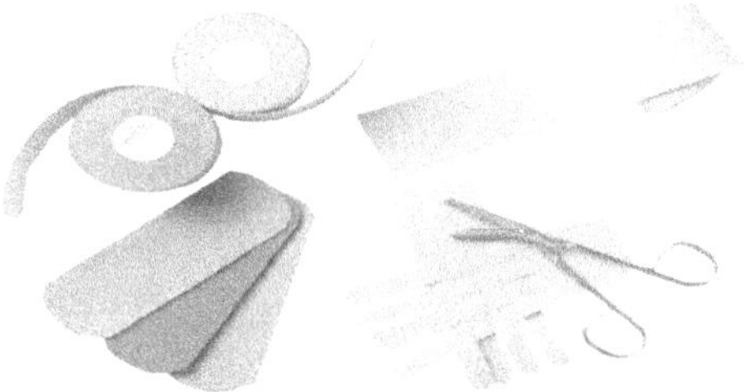

It is important to choose recommended gear that is appropriate for your fitness level, health status, and personal goals. It is also important to consult with a doctor or physical therapist before starting a new workout routine to determine what recommended gear is appropriate for your individual needs.

Safety Tips

Safety is a top priority for seniors during exercise, as they are at a higher risk for injury due to age-related factors such as decreased flexibility, balance, and strength. Here are some safety tips for seniors during exercise:

1. Consult a doctor or physical therapist: Before starting a new workout routine, it is important to consult with a doctor or physical therapist to determine what exercises are appropriate and safe for your individual needs and health status.
2. Start slowly: Gradually increasing the intensity and duration of exercise can help reduce the risk of injury and allow the body to adapt to the new physical demands.
3. Warm up: Warming up before exercise can help prepare the body for physical activity and reduce the risk of injury.
4. Use proper form: Proper form is important to reduce the risk of injury and ensure that exercises are effective. It is recommended to seek guidance from a personal trainer or physical therapist to learn proper form.
5. Wear comfortable clothing and shoes: Wearing comfortable clothing and shoes can help prevent injury and provide support and stability during exercise.
6. Stay hydrated: Staying hydrated before, during, and after exercise can help prevent dehydration and improve overall physical performance.
7. Listen to your body: Pay attention to your body and stop if you experience pain, discomfort, or any other symptoms that could indicate injury or over-exertion.

CHAPTER 5

Motivation and Mindset

Motivation and mindset play a critical role in exercise and physical activity for seniors. Here are some tips for maintaining a positive motivation and mindset during exercise:

Setting Goals

Setting goals is an important step in starting and maintaining an exercise routine for seniors. Here are some tips for setting goals:

1. **Be specific:** Make sure your goals are specific, measurable, and achievable. For example, instead of saying "I want to exercise more," set a goal to "exercise for 30 minutes, three times a week."
2. **Make them realistic:** Make sure your goals are achievable and realistic. Starting with small, manageable goals can help build confidence and motivation to continue.
3. **Set short-term and long-term goals:** Setting both short-term and long-term goals can help keep you motivated and focused on the bigger picture.
4. **Write down your goals:** Writing down your goals can help make them more concrete and help you track progress.
5. **Review and adjust your goals:** Reviewing and adjusting your goals as needed can help you stay on track and maintain motivation.

Staying Motivated

Staying motivated can be challenging, especially when it comes to exercise. Here are some tips for staying motivated during exercise:

1. Find activities you enjoy: Doing activities you enjoy can increase motivation and reduce the risk of boredom and burnout.
2. Exercise with a partner or group: Exercising with others can provide social support, accountability, and encouragement, making it easier to stay motivated.
3. Track progress: Tracking progress can help seniors see the progress they are making and provide a sense of accomplishment and motivation.
4. Reward yourself: Rewarding yourself for meeting fitness goals can increase motivation and provide a positive reinforcement.
5. Focus on the positive: Focusing on the positive aspects of exercise, such as improved health, increased energy, and improved mood, can help maintain motivation.
6. Find an exercise routine that fits into your lifestyle: Finding an exercise routine that fits into your lifestyle can make it easier to stick to a routine and maintain motivation.
7. Stay flexible: Staying flexible and adjusting your exercise routine as needed can help prevent boredom and maintain motivation.

Overcoming Challenges

Overcoming challenges can be a key factor in maintaining an exercise routine for seniors. Here are some tips for overcoming challenges:

1. Find alternative solutions: If an exercise is too challenging, find alternative solutions that are more manageable.

2. Start slowly and gradually increase intensity: Starting slowly and gradually increasing intensity can help prevent injury and increase motivation.

3. Seek support: Seeking support from friends, family, or a healthcare professional can provide encouragement and accountability, making it easier to overcome challenges.

4. Stay flexible: Staying flexible and adjusting your exercise routine as needed can help prevent boredom and overcome challenges.

5. Use proper equipment: Using proper equipment, such as proper shoes and supportive devices, can help prevent injury and overcome physical challenges.

6. Focus on progress: Focusing on progress, rather than perfection, can help seniors overcome challenges and maintain motivation.

7. Stay positive: Staying positive and focusing on the benefits of exercise can help seniors overcome challenges and maintain motivation.

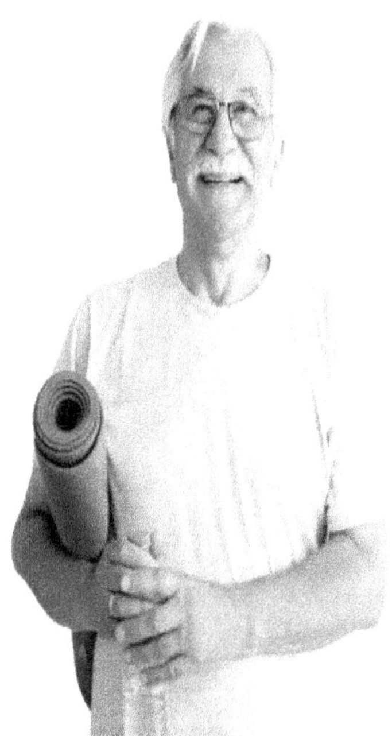

CONCLUSION

Exercise is important for seniors to maintain a healthy lifestyle and improve physical and mental health. Aerobic exercise, strength training, balance and flexibility, low-impact workouts, water exercise, yoga and Pilates, and customized workouts can all provide benefits for seniors.

Safety considerations, such as proper warm-up, cooling down, and using proper equipment, should always be taken into account. Setting goals, staying motivated, and overcoming challenges are also important for maintaining a successful exercise routine. With the right mindset and dedication, seniors can achieve their fitness goals and lead a healthy and active lifestyle.

Exercise is essential for seniors to maintain their health and well-being. Here are some of the key benefits of exercise for seniors:

1. Improved physical health: Exercise helps seniors maintain strength, flexibility, and balance, reducing the risk of falls and other injuries.
2. Enhanced mental health: Exercise can improve mood, reduce stress, and increase cognitive function in seniors.
3. Increased independence: Regular exercise can help seniors maintain independence and reduce the need for assistance.
4. Better sleep: Exercise can improve sleep quality and duration for seniors.
5. Better overall quality of life: Exercise can improve overall health and well-being, leading to a higher quality of life.
6. Reduced risk of chronic disease: Regular exercise can help reduce the risk of chronic diseases such as heart disease, diabetes, and osteoporosis.
7. Increased energy: Exercise can increase energy levels, making it easier to complete daily tasks.

Exercise is a vital aspect of maintaining a healthy lifestyle for seniors.

 From improved physical and mental health, to increased independence and reduced risk of chronic diseases, the benefits of exercise are numerous. With the right mindset, motivation, and safety considerations in mind, seniors can achieve their fitness goals and enjoy a more fulfilling and active lifestyle.

Whether it's through aerobics, strength training, balance and flexibility, low-impact workouts, water exercise, yoga and Pilates, or customized routines, exercise is an important aspect of a healthy lifestyle for seniors. By incorporating exercise into their daily routine, seniors can reap the numerous benefits and lead a healthier and more active life

It's never too late to start an exercise routine and reap the numerous benefits it brings. Staying active is crucial for seniors to maintain physical and mental health and independence. Exercise can be fun, challenging, and rewarding, and it's a great way to stay engaged with friends and community.

So, don't be intimidated, start small and gradually increase your activity level. With the right motivation, mindset, and support, you can achieve your fitness goals and enjoy a healthier and more active lifestyle. Remember, staying active is essential for overall health and well-being, so don't wait any longer, start your exercise journey today!